NUTRITION FOR A HEALTHY LIFE

A GUIDE TO HEALTHY EATING AND IMPROVING YOUR QUALITY OF LIFE

BY

MICHAEL DALE

Table Of Contents

Introduction

Simply said, the body's two distinct and intricate processes for generating energy are significantly different from one another. The two-energy style depends on one another for support because energy is essential to human activity and survival. You can learn which foods in this book will give you the most energy.

We often make the decision to start a health and fitness programme with enthusiasm and perhaps a lot of hype, but after the first week, everything starts to fizzle out. Why do we not follow through with the diet plans, morning jog plans, and fitness plans we make?

What can we do, for our own sakes as well as the sakes of others who depend on us, to ensure that we continue with our plans?

Do you eat to satisfy your hunger or to satisfy your taste buds? Or do you eat in order to have more control over your life? This book demonstrates how focusing on eating properly may greatly improve your quality of life.

CHAPTER 1

THE FUNDAMENTALS

Numerous actions or processes that are frequently taken for granted, such as daily activities, exercise, and the maintenance of growth, require energy. Both of the energy systems share these.

Rarely do any health and exercise plans in the modern world actually work. What is the cause of their alarmingly high failure rate? Two decades ago, the globe was healthier than it is today. This is largely related to people's changing eating patterns.

The Fundamentals

The aerobic system is the main and first energy system to be used. This system puts a lot of demands on the body as a whole and needs oxygen to power the muscles. Due to the concomitant rise in heart rate, this requirement typically causes an increase in the rate, depth, and blood supply.

The body's system naturally switches to the anaerobic energy system when it needs more energy than it can supply because it demands more oxygen than usual. This system has the ability to generate energy without using oxygen.

All of this energy is produced through appropriate or sensible food consumption. The types of energy levels that each person can produce depend on the foods consumed. When all available energy sources have been used up, muscle weariness usually sets in for a variety of reasons, the most compelling one being the kinds of foods that have been ingested.

It is important to note the foods that develop or boost the energy generating sources because there are many food categories that offer different health benefits for the human body system. The person should be able to select the appropriate foods with the use of this knowledge.

The anaerobic system releases energy from nutrients stored in the body, typically during severe activity bouts, whereas the aerobic system breaks down the carbs, fatty acids, and amino acids in the foods consumed. If we hear about diet or exercise failures all around us, it's usually not their fault.

Those who made a big deal about following through on these plans, told all their friends and coworkers about them, and then failed to do so, are usually to blame. Naturally, those who drop out of a fitness or diet programme midway do not perceive the benefits, and everyone blames the programme.

What the world needs right now is motivation, not a brand-new diet or exercise regimen. To carry out whatever strategy they have chosen all the way through, the right mindset is required.

If they can accomplish that, the majority of health problems linked to lifestyle choices will become obsolete. The best part is that we don't need to travel far to find this drive. We just need to look inside and use the motivation that is already inside of us.

People wouldn't have dreamed of buying whatever junk food they could acquire to feed their faces a generation ago. Today, we act in that manner extremely casually. When someone says, "I'm hungry," they typically mean, "I want a burger or a hot dog, perhaps with crackers and some coke." Furthermore, saying "I'm on a diet" actually means "I'm taking a chemical-laden tablet that will snuff out my hunger and deprive my body of vitamins." Actually, it makes no sense that we are currently dealing with so many health difficulties.

Our health is a reflection of the foods we eat. The unfortunate state in which we find ourselves is not an issue that only affects one person. Everyone in the world eats improperly. By the year 2023, eight out of ten people in the US will be overweight, up from the current figure of six out of ten.

Are we really considering this? We're not. You're probably snacking on a bag of chips while reading this book. Do you realise that the money you spent on that package, which contains some of the most dangerous substances known to man, might have instead been used to feed a malnourished child in Rwanda?

But it goes beyond simply being charitable. It also pertains to us. Yes, we must be self-centered. Are we on the verge of a catastrophe with such horrifying health statistics? We definitely aren't eating properly. We must be ready for any excess baggage that comes with obesity and the various illnesses it leaves behind.

Therefore, keep in mind that criticism isn't likely coming because a programme is unstable the next time you find it has failed or is drawing a lot of negative attention. Most often, it's because people had good intentions at first but didn't adhere to the programme as strictly as they should have.

CHAPTER 2

YOUR PERSPECTIVE ON FOOD

Even more important than a trainer or a doctor, your personal motivation is what you need to keep your health and fitness programme going. To carefully examine the situation, you must be committed. You are overweight, therefore you want to lose a few pounds.

If you don't take the necessary steps to have the proper diet and to adhere to your regular exercise schedule, no gym instructor from anywhere in the world will be able to help you. No doctor will be able to help you, even if you are unwell and seeking treatment, if you are not committed to adhering to the recommended course of action, whether that involves taking medication at the recommended time or avoiding certain foods.

Your Attitude

So far, we have drastically departed from our normal dietary patterns. Things won't get better unless we assess the situation and take action on our own.

The most important factor is awareness. We must educate ourselves about which foods are healthy for us and which are not. We need to go back to our training to understand what nutrients, and in what quantities, your body actually needs.

Then, to ensure that we eat healthily, we must create a diet plan for both ourselves and our loved ones. We need to eat fewer foods that are bad for us—sugars, fats, and carbohydrates are things we don't really need—while increasing the amounts of foods that may be good for our health.

I realise that this does sound a bit overly preachy. However, that is the only break we have. We'll never get better as long as we keep eating Oreos. Still, there is hope. There are many things that are just as delicious as those horrible junk foods, but we are just learning about them, so there is still hope.

These are the foods we don't yet know about; we probably don't like them, or we don't know how to prepare them, but a healthy cookbook may allow you to understand several intriguing ways to cook healthily. You can create some incredibly delectable healthy recipes even with the same type of diet you now follow. All of that is definitely feasible. You can significantly alter your eating patterns while also paying attention to your palate.

The truth is that the weight loss industry has significantly contributed to the decline of the advanced human race. Atkins, Jenny Craig, Zone, and Medi-fast must continue to be sold, thus the media never informs you of how you can take matters into your own hands.

They flash before-and-after photos of a person with a foot-long sub and then a man with six pack abs, telling us that the diet was what allowed for that transformation. The truth is that we could very easily achieve that as well, without having to spend thousands of dollars on such diets, if we were to get our act together. What must we do, then?

Two things in general: -Regulate our intake. Engage in some physical activity.

Is it a difficult task to complete now? Don't we owe that to our bodies, which have been so helpful to us for so long? Don't we owe that to our family members and ourselves?

CHAPTER 3

WHOLE GRAINS AND HONEY

Honey has been shown to be the energy circle's sole sustaining force over time. It continues to be unparalleled in its ability to produce energy while also benefiting the human body in other ways. The most natural source of energy is honey. In addition to acting as a powerful immune system booster, it also functions as a natural cure for a wide range of diseases.

The natural flow of a human being's daily life cycle depends heavily on energy. Finding reliable and nutritious energy sources is crucial for maintaining your health and happiness.

A Potent Pair

Honey’s inherent advantages have long been understood and accepted. Honey is also a natural source of carbohydrates, which are an energy source for enhancing performance, endurance, and lowering levels of muscular tiredness. Honey also has a nice taste.

For athletes, this is very helpful. The honey's sugar content aids in avoiding weariness both during physical activity and throughout sports enthusiasts' training sessions. Glucose and fructose, which make up these sugars, have sepa rate but complementary roles.

The honey's glucose component often absorbs more quickly and provides an immediate energy boost, whilst the fructose works more slowly and provides a longer-lasting and more sustained energy release. Honey has been shown to assist in maintaining steady blood sugar levels in the body when it comes to this issue.

Consuming honey is not a particularly tough activity because it is a tasty food item and is natural in its form. In general, people of all ages are eager to consume honey in any of its auxiliary forms. Even little youngsters like it.

Consuming honey is not a particularly tough activity because it is a tasty food item and is natural in its form. In general, people of all ages are eager to consume honey in any of its auxiliary forms. Even little youngsters like it.

A modest amount of honey consumed each day gives kids the energy they need to handle the physical demands of their everyday activities at school and in sports.

Even for adults, a tiny amount of honey every day can help maintain a high level of energy throughout a busy workday. One approach to making a tasty snack is to make sandwiches with honey and other ingredients.

Another delicious breakfast option is to spread honey on a slice of freshly baked bread. It is recommended to use honey in place of sugar when making beverages. The majority of people in today's society seek quick fixes for their energy-boosting requirements, which typically come in the form of unhealthy sports drinks, coffee, and processed carbs like sugar and white bread.

Although these give the desired boost in energy, it should be noted that this energy is relatively fleeting and the fatigue that follows is typically felt more sharply. As a result, consuming any form of whole grain is not only a better option, but also much healthier.

Whole grains offer energy that is present in a more complex form and breaks down gradually over time. This then establishes the foundation for maintaining energy levels for longer periods of time.

Whole grains have a variety of healthy components because of their more complex makeup, including fibre and a wealth of phytonutrients, minerals, and vitamins. Any dish's flavour is frequently finished off or improved by the addition of whole grain ingredients. There are many different types of whole grains, including wheat, oat, barley, maize, brown rice, faro, spelt, emmer, einkorn, rye, millet, buckwheat, and many more. These can then be used to create a variety of additional products, including teff flour, whole wheat flour, whole wheat bread, whole wheat pasta, rolled oats or oat groats, triticale flour, popcorn, and whole wheat flour.

Consistently eating whole grains can help control weight, lower cholesterol levels, defend against several types of cancer, and reduce the risk of heart disease. It is important to distinguish whole grains from their inferior and refined “relatives.” Even though refined grains offer some advantages, whole grain substitutes are always preferable.

CHAPTER 4

LEAN MEAT AND NUTS

For both human and animal use, nuts are a vital source of nutrition. Given its abundance of essential nutrients, it can be consumed raw, cooked, or as a supplement to already prepared foods. Despite the fact that a nut is typically thought of as a hard-shelled fruit, the nut family actually includes a wide range of other foods.

While different kinds of meat typically contribute to a diversity of flavours, the healthiest kind is the one that contains the most lean meat. It is undeniable that meats with a substantial level of fat are a gourmet treat, but it is wise to take the time to learn about the advantages of eating lean meats for health reasons.

Healthy Oils And Proteins

It is now widely known that nuts significantly aid in keeping many illnesses under control or preventing them altogether.

For instance, nuts have been shown to be able to prevent the development of coronary heart disease, even in

people who have a long line of relatives who have the condition.

The body's blood cholesterol levels have been shown to decrease after consuming nuts like almonds and walnuts. For those with issues with insulin resistance, such as diabetics, nuts are also strongly advised.

Another better option is to satisfy cravings with almonds rather than junk food. Another benefit of choosing nuts as a healthier choice is that they contain vital fatty acids. Another benefit of having nuts on hand as snacks is that they are nutritious and may be eaten in their raw form.

Due to their delayed burn properties, which aid in maintaining stable blood sugar levels, almonds are frequently used to balance blood lipids. The almond is a well-liked addition to the monotonous diet of the majority of Mediterranean people because it is rich in a variety of different nutrients.

Another healthy nut is the Brazil nut, which has its own advantages when eaten in moderation. The Brazil nut, which is well-known for having omega-3 fatty acids, is also a strong source of calcium.

Another very well-liked nut that is frequently eaten as a salted snack is the cashew nut. However, as it is already a fairly savoury nut on its own, it would be a much healthier food product without the addition of salt. These nuts are processed into oils in several regions of the world.

The selection procedure should be carried out with some understanding because relying just on what the unaided eye can see is insufficient. The following beef cuts should generally be considered lean: round, chuck, sirloin, and tenderloin. Tenderloin, loin chops, and legs would be considered lean meats from pork or lamb. The chicken's breast portion without the skin would be the leanest part.

There are many reasons why people choose to omit meat from their diets, but there is no proof that doing so is either healthy or appropriate for everyone.

The choice of meats that would make consumption healthy, and this would typically mean meats with reduced fat content, is the crucial factor to keep in mind in this situation. Compared to red meat, white meat has far less fat, but it is by no means deficient in fat. Consuming lean meats has a significant and well-rounded nutritional benefit.

The protein content of lean meats is typically higher and purer, which is a crucial component of the sustenance and development of every cell's fundamental structural and functional advancement.

Essential amino acids, notably sulphur amino acids, are also abundant in lean meats.
When compared to digestion rates, animal proteins function more quickly than those found
in beans and whole grains.

Additionally, a good source of iron is lean meat. Due to the gradual nature of iron deficiency, it frequently goes undetected until anaemia has set in.

CHAPTER 5

THE ADVANTAGES

You have every reason in the world to keep eating well after reading this. Let's start discussing the topic right away.

BENEFITS

Your Health Improves

Even if we had a library of books on the benefits of healthy eating, they wouldn't fully describe the benefits that are actually there. The main benefit is that you gain control over your weight.

- By choosing healthy foods, you also ensure that your digestive and immune systems, as well as other metabolic processes, continue to operate as intended. Additionally, you are guarded against a range of chronic illnesses, including diabetes and conditions related to the heart, including high blood pressure and coronary artery disease.

Additional Savings

You can save a lot of money by eating healthfully. Your grocery expenses drop significantly, and if credit card debt is already a problem for you, you avoid adding to it. Additionally, you avoid spending a fortune on any medical costs that may arise as a result of your food bingeing behaviour.

Your Body Contains Fewer Toxins

Given the presence of synthetic chemicals in modern diets, many of them are poisonous. One of the fundamental tenets of eating properly is that you shouldn't eat anything that is man-made, so when you try to eat right, you are far less likely to introduce these poisons into your body.

Additionally, by eating less, you'll be able to cut back on vices like smoking and drunkenness. Beer is nearly always associated with a night out with the guys. You won't need as much beer if you eat less. Similar to this, you won't want to have your customary one or more cigarettes after every meal.

More Active Lifestyle

You'll discover that your ability to work much more effectively increases as a result of better eating habits. Your life can be more productive as a result of your increased ability to work out, travel, play, and work.

Don't you think that is better than being a slob and spending the entire day on the couch? Additionally, you have more opportunities to interact with friends and family, which unquestionably improves your quality of life.

Decent Social Life

Forget about "fat fetishism." Overweight people don't look good. Weight in the wrong areas of the body is strongly stigmatised in society. Your extra weight can actually hinder your ability to locate a companion. Not only that, but those who have trouble controlling their eating and weight are viewed negatively by society as having trouble controlling their basic desires.

There is this kind of psychology, but very few people will talk about it. You'll find that these problems go away when you eat properly.

Conclusions

Today's market offers a variety of well-liked diets, but the majority of them are harmful and occasionally even

dangerous. This will outline how to maintain a balanced, nutritious diet for life and steer clear of bad diets.

Find out how many calories your body needs each day to function.

Depending on your metabolism and level of physical activity, this number could vary greatly. Your daily caloric intake should remain at around 2000 calories for men and 1500 calories for women if you're the type of person who gains 10 pounds after just smelling a slice of pizza.

Additionally, your body mass affects this: For naturally bigger people, more calories are suitable, and for smaller people, fewer calories are. You may want to boost your daily calorie intake by 1000–2000 calories, a little less for women, if you're the type of person who can eat without gaining weight or you're physically active.

Eat fatty foods without fear.

For your body to function properly, you must consume fat from food. But it's important to choose the right kinds of fat: The majority of animal fats and a few vegetable oils are high in the LDL (bad) cholesterol-raising kind of fat.

Contrary to popular opinion, eating cholesterol doesn't always increase your body's level of cholesterol. Your body will eliminate additional cholesterol if you give it the right resources. You should strive to routinely take monounsaturated fatty acids, which are those tools. Olive oil, almonds, fish oil, and various seed oils are foods that are high in monounsaturated fatty acids.

Consume a lot of the right kinds of carbohydrates.

Since carbohydrates are your body's primary source of energy, you must consume foods high in carbohydrates. The secret is to choose the right carbs. Sugar and refined wheat are examples of simple carbohydrates that are rapidly absorbed by the body.

This produces a sort of carb overflow, and your body generates massive amounts of insulin to counteract the overload. In addition to harming your heart, too much insulin also promotes weight growth.

Consume lots of carbohydrates, but choose those that the body can absorb gradually, such as whole-grain flour, vegetables, oats, and unprocessed grains.

Start the day with a larger meal.

Towards the end of the evening, your metabolism slows down and becomes less effective at breaking down food. As a result, less of the meal's nutritional value will be absorbed by your body and more of the food's energy will be stored as fat.

Consider having a medium-sized breakfast, a large lunch, and a small dinner. Better yet, try eating 4-6 small meals throughout the course of your day.

Give yourself a cheat meal.

Cheating involves indulging in a food you actually love once a week rather than bingeing on all the wrong foods every week. Have a few slices of pizza on Sundays or a giant slice of double chocolate cake on Saturdays..

This cheat meal is beneficial to your health in a number of ways and will help you persist with the diet modification. Cheat meals are permitted on special occasions like family birthdays.

Establish a slow-eating routine.

With fewer calories, it will make you feel full and prevent obesity and all of its negative effects.

Drink a lot of water.

Your skin will thank you, you'll feel more awake and energised, and you'll eat less because it makes you feel fuller. If you reduce your soda use, water will be much better for you.

www.ingramcontent.com/pod-product-compliance
Lightning Source LLC
LaVergne TN
LVHW020538160826
845677LV00015B/4137